Contents

Foreword

Until recently, celiac disease was considered a medical curiosity. Most physicians, registered dietitians, and other health care professionals knew little about the disease and spent little time explaining it to patients. Likewise, discussion of the gluten-free diet was limited. Only a few people required this diet, and health care providers usually told those who did to simply avoid wheat, rye, barley, and oats.

In the past decades, however, we have learned a phenomenal amount about celiac disease and other gluten-related disorders. Even in the eight years since the last edition of the *Celiac Disease Nutrition Guide* was published, our knowledge has expanded. We now recognize that celiac disease is one of the most common autoimmune diseases, affecting around 1% of most populations, and we know that there are large groups of people without celiac disease who also seem to benefit from a gluten-free or gluten-restricted diet. Well-designed studies in both the United States and Europe have shown that the true prevalence of celiac disease is much higher today than it was 50 years ago, and this trend does not show signs of slowing down. Notably, the rising rates of celiac disease coincide with increases in the incidence of other chronic inflammatory disorders, such as type 1 diabetes and inflammatory bowel disease.

Generations born today in North America may have upwards of a 2% to 3% lifetime risk of celiac disease. Furthermore, in the coming decades, an unknown number of people will follow a gluten-free or gluten-restricted diet for conditions other than celiac disease, such as autism, non-celiac gluten sensitivity, and irritable bowel syndrome. All told, an estimated 5 million to 10 million people in the United States may need to follow a gluten-free diet in the coming years. As a comparison, fewer than 1 million people in the United States have type 1 diabetes.

A number of novel nondietary therapies are currently being developed for celiac disease. However, it is highly unlikely that any of these treatments will replace the need for a strict, balanced gluten-free diet. With this in mind, I am very enthusiastic about the release of the Third Edition of the *Celiac Disease Nutrition Guide*. This booklet is an extremely valuable reference, which accurately explains celiac disease and other gluten-related disorders. It provides a solid foundation for the lifestyle changes that these diagnoses require. I congratulate the author, Tricia Thompson, and the Academy of Nutrition and Dietetics on this work and recommend it without reservation to individuals and families beginning a gluten-free diet.

To your health,

Daniel A. Leffler, MD, MS
Director of Research at the Celiac Center
Beth Israel Deaconess Medical Center
Associate Professor of Medicine
Harvard Medical School

If you are reading this book, it is likely that you or a loved one has been diagnosed with celiac disease, dermatitis herpetiformis, or non-celiac gluten sensitivity (NCGS). Learning what foods to avoid and what to eat is a key part of your treatment.

This book focuses on the gluten-free diet used to manage celiac disease. However, the nutrition advice can also help people with dermatitis herpetiformis or NCGS. Before we discuss the details of the gluten-free diet, let's start by learning the basics about gluten and each of these conditions.

> **Note:** If you have **not** already been diagnosed with celiac disease, dermatitis herpetiformis, or NCGS, see your doctor before you start a gluten-free diet. The diagnosis of celiac disease is based on blood tests and a biopsy of the small intestine. If you start a gluten-free diet before testing, the test results may not lead to an accurate diagnosis.

What Is Gluten?

Gluten is the common name for the proteins (**prolamins** and **glutelins**) in wheat, barley, and rye that must not be eaten on a gluten-free diet. Strictly speaking, however, gluten is a protein found only in wheat.

> **Note**: The word "gluten" is sometimes used as a general term to describe prolamins found in many grains, including corn. This is why you may see or hear the term "corn gluten." Corn gluten is fine for you to eat.

What Are Promalins?

Wheat prolamins are called **gliadin**. Barley prolamins are **hordein**. Rye prolamins are **secalin**. These three types of prolamins are harmful to people with celiac disease.

Prolamins from other grains do not harm people with celiac disease. For example, orzenin (the prolamin in rice) and zein (the prolamin in corn) are safe for people with celiac disease to eat.

What Are Glutelins?

Glutelins are another type of protein found in grains. The glutelins of wheat, barley, and rye are also harmful to people with celiac disease.

What Is Celiac Disease?

Celiac disease is a type of autoimmune disease that is genetically inherited. An **autoimmune disease** is a condition where the immune system damages the body in response to something it views as harmful.

With celiac disease, your immune system views gluten as harmful. When you eat gluten, your immune system causes inflammation and damages your small intestine.

Because of this damage, the small intestine cannot fully absorb nutrients, including carbohydrates, proteins, fats, vitamins, and minerals. The side effects can include:

- Weight loss
- Tiredness
- Vitamin and mineral deficiencies (for example, deficiencies of iron, folate, calcium, or fat-soluble vitamins)
- Iron-deficiency anemia
- Bone disease
- Gastrointestinal symptoms, including diarrhea, constipation, bloating, and excess gas

Note: Not everyone with celiac disease will experience gastrointestinal symptoms.

What Is Dermatitis Herpetiformis?

Dermatitis herpetiformis is a type of celiac disease that affects the skin. When people with dermatitis herpetiformis eat gluten, they get a painful rash. The reaction to gluten also damages the small intestine of most people with this condition. A skin biopsy and blood tests are used to diagnose dermatitis herpetiformis.

What Is Non-Celiac Gluten Sensitivity?

Non-celiac gluten sensitivity (NCGS) refers to another type of response to gluten, which is not an allergy or autoimmune disease. People with NCGS may have gastrointestinal symptoms similar to those experienced by people with celiac disease.

There are currently no tests to diagnose NCGS. A person may receive an NCGS diagnosis once his or her doctor rules out celiac disease and other conditions.

It is important to note that there is much that we do not know about NCGS. Eating certain carbohydrates as well as parts of wheat (other than gluten) may play a role in symptoms.

What Is a Gluten-Free Diet?

Celiac disease, dermatitis herpetiformis, and NCGS are all considered to be gluten-related disorders. People with these disorders should follow a lifelong gluten-free diet, strictly avoiding wheat, rye, and barley proteins.

All other grain proteins (with the possible exception of oats) are considered safe to eat. For more information on oats, see page 36 in the Frequently Asked Questions section of this booklet.

A gluten-free diet allows the intestine to heal and improves gastrointestinal symptoms, such as diarrhea, constipation, excess gas, and bloating. The gluten-free diet may also help prevent conditions that can be caused by **long-term** untreated celiac disease, such as lymphoma (a cancer of the lymph tissue) and osteoporosis (the chronic loss of bone mass).

Grains to Avoid

Do **not** eat these grains when following a gluten-free diet:

- **Wheat**, including all varieties, such as spelt; khorasan; einkorn; emmer; and most forms, such as wheat starch (unless labeled gluten-free), wheat flours (for example, semolina), wheat bran, wheat germ, cracked wheat, and hydrolyzed wheat protein
- **Rye**
- **Barley**, including most forms, such as malt, malt flavoring, and malt extract
- **Crossbred varieties of gluten-containing grains**, such as triticale (a cross between wheat and rye)
- **Oats** that are **not** labeled gluten-free

Grains That Are Considered Safe

You can safely eat these grains as part of a gluten-free diet:

- Amaranth
- Buckwheat
- Corn
- Millet
- Oats (labeled gluten-free only)
- Quinoa
- Rice
- Sorghum
- Tef (or teff)
- Wild rice

Flours and starches used in gluten-free products are also made from arrowroot, beans, cassava, flax, lentils, nuts, peas, potato, sago, seeds, soy, tapioca, and yucca.

> **Note**: Whenever possible, buy naturally gluten-free grains, flours, and starches that are **labeled** gluten-free. Compared to similar products that are not labeled gluten-free, these products are less likely to have come into cross-contact with wheat, barley, or rye. Read more about cross-contact on page 13.

Treatment Beyond the Gluten-Free Diet

After diagnosis of celiac disease, your doctor may evaluate and treat you for associated conditions, such as other autoimmune diseases, anemia, or bone disease.

Treatment of dermatitis herpetiformis may include topical medications in addition to the gluten-free diet. With these treatments, both the skin and intestine can heal.

What to Look for on a Food Label

Most of the information you need to follow a gluten-free diet can be found on food labels. To stay safe, read **all** food labels and make choices that are gluten-free.

Start by looking for the words **gluten-free**. When a food is labeled gluten-free, you may include it in your diet. (For more information on what the term "gluten-free" means when it is printed on a food label, see page 7.)

When a product is **not** labeled gluten-free, you need to look for the following six words in the ingredients list:

1. Wheat
2. Rye
3. Barley
4. Oats
5. Malt (unless a gluten-free source is named, such as corn malt)
6. Brewer's yeast

Do **not** eat foods that have any of these six words in the ingredients list. You also should **not** eat foods if you see the words **"Contains Wheat"** next to the ingredients list, unless the food is labeled gluten-free. (See page 9 for more information on Contains statements.)

For almost all foods that are not labeled gluten-free, you need to check labels for only the six ingredients listed above. This is because most foods are required to follow labeling rules set by the U.S. Food and Drug Administration (FDA).

However, the labeling rules are a bit different for foods regulated by the U.S. Department of Agriculture (USDA). These foods include:
- Meat products (for example, hot dogs)
- Poultry products (for example, seasoned turkey breast)
- Egg products (for example, some liquid egg products)
- Mixed food products that contain certain amounts of meat or poultry (for example, some stews and some chili)

When a food product is regulated by the USDA and is **not** labeled gluten-free, you need to check the label for **nine** terms (the same six listed on page 5, plus three more):
1. Wheat
2. Rye
3. Barley
4. Oats
5. Malt (unless a gluten-free source is named, such as corn malt)
6. Brewer's yeast
7. Dextrin
8. Modified food starch
9. Starch

Do **not** eat a USDA-regulated food that lists any of the first six ingredients or says "Contains Wheat" on the label. Also, do **not** eat a USDA-regulated food if it lists any of the last three ingredients, unless the source of the ingredient is provided and that source is not wheat, rye, or barley (for example, cornstarch).

Read more about USDA-regulated foods on page 8. Advice for reading labels on alcoholic beverages is also found on page 8. Go to pages 13 and 14 for information about what to look for on supplement and medication labels.

> **Note**: If you have a question about an ingredient, contact the manufacturer. Contact information is generally provided on product packaging.

What Does "Gluten-Free" Mean?

As we've noted, when you see the words "gluten-free" on a food label, you know you can choose that food. But what exactly does the term "gluten-free" mean? Let's look at how it is defined in the labeling rules of three U.S. government agencies: the FDA, the USDA, and the TTB (Alcohol and Tobacco Tax and Trade Bureau).

Gluten-Free Labeling of FDA-Regulated Foods

The FDA published the final rule for the labeling of food as gluten-free on August 5, 2013. Under this rule, gluten-free labeling is voluntary. In other words, food manufacturers are not required to use the term "gluten-free" on labels of foods that meet the FDA definition of gluten-free. However, when a food is labeled "gluten-free," it must meet the FDA's requirements.

The FDA rule applies to the labeling of packaged foods (including dietary supplements) regulated by the FDA. It does not apply to pet foods, cosmetics, prescription and nonprescription drugs, foods regulated by the USDA, or beverages regulated by the TTB.

Under the FDA rule, a food can be labeled gluten-free when the unavoidable presence of gluten in the food is less than 20 parts per million (ppm). To be labeled gluten-free, the food must:

- Be naturally gluten-free, such as bottled water or a bag of raw carrots, **or**
- Meet **both** of the following criteria:
  - ° The food does **not** contain an ingredient that is a gluten-containing grain (for example, wheat).
  - ° The food does **not** contain an ingredient derived from a gluten-containing grain that has not been processed to remove gluten (for example, wheat flour).

What Does "Parts per Million" (ppm) Mean?

Parts per million is a proportion that indicates how many parts out of 1 million parts are gluten. In 1 kilogram of food, 20 ppm equals 20 milligrams of gluten (because 1 kilogram contains 1 million milligrams).

A gluten-free food **may** contain an ingredient derived from a gluten-containing grain that has been processed to remove gluten (for example, wheat starch), as long as use of that ingredient in the food does **not** cause the food to contain 20 or more ppm of gluten.

Under this rule, foods labeled "no gluten," "free of gluten," and "without gluten" must meet the same criteria as foods labeled "gluten-free."

Gluten-Free Labeling of USDA-Regulated Foods

The USDA does not plan to issue a rule to define "gluten-free" on the labels of the foods it regulates. However, the USDA has stated that meat, poultry, and egg product manufacturers will need to follow FDA labeling rules if they choose to label a product gluten-free. The USDA plans to publish its official position on its website now that the final FDA rule has been released.

Gluten-Free Labeling of TTB-Regulated Alcoholic Beverages

The TTB regulates almost all alcoholic beverages **except:**
- Beer and other malt beverages made without either malted barley or hops
- Wines with less than 7% alcohol by volume

These exceptions are regulated by the FDA.

In May 2012, the TTB issued an interim policy on the labeling of alcoholic beverages under its jurisdiction. Under this policy, a TTB-regulated alcoholic beverage may be labeled gluten-free if:
- It is made without any gluten-containing grains or ingredients derived from these grains (for example, barley malt).
- Producers can ensure that the raw ingredients and finished product (among other things) are **not** cross-contaminated with gluten.

For more information on alcoholic beverages, see the final Frequently Asked Question on page 37.

> ## The Regulation of Beer and Gluten-Free Labeling
>
> Beer regulated by the TTB may not be labeled gluten-free.
> The FDA regulates beers made using a substitute for malted
> barley. These beers may be labeled gluten-free if they meet all
> FDA labeling criteria.

Food Allergen Labeling

In addition to the rules about gluten-free labeling, there is another U.S.
labeling rule that can help people with celiac disease identify foods they
should avoid: the **Food Allergen Labeling and Consumer Protection
Act of 2004 (FALCPA)**.

What Does FALCPA Require?

Under FALCPA, if an ingredient in an FDA-regulated packaged food
product contains protein from wheat, the word "wheat" must be clearly
stated on the food label, either in the ingredients list (for example, wheat
flour) or in a separate Contains statement (for example, Contains Wheat).

FALCPA applies to **all** ingredients, including modified food starch, dextrin, flavorings, colorings, and incidental additives. In addition, if a spice
blend or seasoning mix includes an ingredient containing wheat protein,
the word "wheat" must be clearly stated on the food label.

> **Note:** Modified food starch and dextrin may be derived from
> wheat, although they are usually made from corn. If they
> contain wheat protein, the word "wheat" will be clearly stated
> in the ingredients list or a Contains statement.

In addition to wheat, FALCPA requires that manufacturers identify seven
other major food allergens in a food product's ingredients list or Contains
statement: milk, eggs, fish, Crustacean shellfish, tree nuts, peanuts, and
soybeans. FALCPA does **not** apply to barley or rye.

The following examples of ingredients lists for enriched spaghetti will give you an idea of what food labels that comply with FALCPA look like.

Example 1

Ingredients: Semolina (wheat), niacin, reduced iron, thiamin mononitrate, riboflavin, folic acid.

Example 2

Ingredients: Semolina, niacin, reduced iron, thiamin mononitrate, riboflavin, folic acid. Contains Wheat.

Food Allergen Labeling of USDA-Regulated Foods

Manufacturers of USDA-regulated foods, such as meat products, poultry products, or egg products, are not required to follow FALCPA. However, almost all manufacturers of USDA-regulated foods voluntarily comply with allergen labeling. There is a very small chance that a USDA-regulated food could include modified food starch, dextrin, or starch derived from wheat but would not use the word "wheat" in the ingredients list or a separate Contains statement.

Gluten-Free Foods That List Wheat Ingredients

Some products are labeled gluten-free but include the word "wheat" in the ingredients list or Contains statement. This labeling may seem odd. However, it is allowed because certain ingredients derived from wheat may be included in foods labeled gluten-free as long as the final food product contains less than 20 ppm of gluten. Examples of such ingredients are wheat starch, modified food starch (wheat), and ingredients that may be made from wheat starch, including dextrin (wheat), maltodextrin (wheat), glucose syrup (wheat), and caramel (wheat).

Under the FDA's gluten-free labeling rule, if a food is labeled gluten-free and also includes the word "wheat" in the ingredients list or Contains statement, the following must be added to the label, "The wheat has been processed to allow this food to meet the Food and Drug Administration requirements for gluten-free foods."

Bottom line: You may include **all** food labeled gluten-free in your diet even when the food includes a Contains statement for wheat.

Food Products and Ingredients Made from Barley

The following food products and ingredients are usually made from barley:
- Beer, ale, porter, stout, and other similar fermented beverages
- Malt
- Malt syrup/malt extract
- Malt beverages
- Malted milk
- Malt vinegar

The foods in this list should **not** be eaten unless they are labeled gluten-free (such as sorghum-based beer) or a grain source other than barley, wheat, or rye is listed on the food label (such as corn malt).

> **Note**: Non-malt vinegars, including cider vinegar, wine vinegar, balsamic vinegar, and distilled vinegar, are safe for people with celiac disease. The single word "vinegar" in an ingredients list means the vinegar was made from apples.

Identifying Processed Foods That May Contain Harmful Grains

Manufacturers may change their products at any time. **To be safe, check the ingredients on the labels of all processed foods not labeled gluten-free every time you shop**. Look carefully for sources of harmful ingredients in food, such as:
- Bouillon cubes
- Brown rice syrup
- Candy
- Cold cuts, hot dogs, salami, sausage

- Communion wafers (altar breads)
- French fries
- Gravies
- Imitation fish
- Matzo and matzo meal
- Rice mixes
- Sauces
- Seasoned tortilla chips or potato chips
- Self-basting turkey
- Soups
- Soy sauce
- Vegetables in sauce

Communion Wafers

Communion wafers are usually made from wheat. However, some gluten-free food manufacturers (for example, Ener-G Foods, Inc.) make wheat-free, gluten-free wafers. Ask your local church if you are allowed to use such a wafer.

The Roman Catholic Church does not allow the use of wheat-free, gluten-free communion wafers to celebrate the Eucharist. However, the Benedictine Sisters of Perpetual Adoration make a wheat-based, low-gluten wafer that conforms to Canon Law.

For more information on communion wafers, see page 21.

Matzo and Matzo Meal

Matzo and matzo meal are usually made from wheat. However, gluten-free matzo made from certified gluten-free oat flour is available from Lakewood Matzoh Bakery. According to the manufacturer website, its matzo is Hamotzi and appropriate for Seder use.

Yehuda brand matzo is made from various gluten-free starches. It is available from various companies, including Amazon (www.amazon.com).

For more information on matzo, see page 21.

Cross-Contact

Cross-contact can occur whenever a gluten-free food comes in contact with a food that contains gluten. The potential for cross-contact exists for all foods, whether they are specially made to be gluten-free or just happen not to contain gluten.

Cross-contact can happen anywhere from the field to the factory. For example, a gluten-free food could be grown next to wheat, barley, or rye, or it could be processed on equipment also used for those grains. **Foods labeled gluten-free must contain less than 20 ppm of gluten, including the gluten from any possible cross-contact.**

Some packaged gluten-free foods are processed in facilities that make only gluten-free foods. However, even if a gluten-free facility is used, ingredients brought into the facility (including naturally gluten-free grains and flours) may be contaminated with gluten. This is one reason why it is so important that manufacturers test all products they label as gluten-free to ensure that the products actually contain less than 20 ppm of gluten.

Packaged gluten-free foods can be produced in facilities that also make gluten-containing foods. These facilities may have a dedicated room or production line for gluten-free products. Other facilities may run gluten-free foods on the same production line as gluten-containing foods. These foods will not necessarily be contaminated with gluten. All manufacturers are required to follow current standards of good manufacturing practice and take steps to lower the risk of cross-contact (such as thorough cleaning of shared equipment).

If you have any questions about how a food product is processed and whether it is tested for gluten, contact the manufacturer.

Choosing Gluten-Free Dietary Supplements

Nonprescription dietary supplements, such as vitamins and minerals, are covered under FALCPA. Therefore, if an ingredient (including a flavoring, coloring, or additive) in a supplement contains wheat protein, the word "wheat" will be listed in either the ingredients list or a Contains statement. Always read the supplement labels, and contact the manufacturer if you have any questions about whether a product is free of gluten-containing ingredients.

Brands of gluten-free vitamin and mineral supplements include Country Life, C-liac Vitality Packs, Freeda, and Pioneer Nutritionals.

Choosing Gluten-Free Medications

Over-the-counter and prescription medications are **not** covered under FALCPA. Be aware that these products may contain fillers or coatings made from gluten-containing grains. More information on gluten-free medications is available at www.glutenfreedrugs.com. See also the Additional Sources of Information in this booklet.

> **Note**: Infant formulas and medical foods are covered under FALCPA. If ingredients in these products contain protein from wheat, the word "wheat" must be clearly listed on the label in either the ingredients list or Contains statement.

Over-the-Counter Medications

Always review the ingredients lists on labels of over-the-counter medications. Ingredients may be separated into active components (ingredients with a healing benefit, such as reducing fever or pain) and inactive ingredients (such as flavoring and coloring). Contact the manufacturer if you have questions about whether a product is free of gluten-containing ingredients.

Prescription Medications

Prescription medications do not usually list ingredients on the label. Talk with your pharmacist, doctor, and/or the manufacturer about whether your medications are free of gluten-containing ingredients.

Where to Find Gluten-Free Foods

Following a gluten-free diet affects the types of grain foods you can eat. The good news is that you can find a wide variety of gluten-free grain products from mail order companies, natural food stores, and even your local grocery store.

> **Remember**: Because of the risk of cross-contact with wheat, barley, or rye, **it is best to buy grain products that are labeled gluten-free whenever possible**. Manufacturers who label their products gluten-free must follow the FDA gluten-free labeling rule.
>
> If you buy grain products that are not labeled gluten-free (which is **not** advised), **always** check labels to make sure they do not include any gluten-containing ingredients.

Gluten-Free Shopping at Your Supermarket

Many supermarkets now carry gluten-free foods. At your supermarket, look in the natural foods section or ask the manager where the gluten-free foods are located. Gluten-free foods may be in one section or spread throughout the store. Also look for shelf tags, which some supermarkets use to help customers find gluten-free products.

Some food manufacturers have changed their products to be gluten-free. Manufacturers also use the gluten-free label for foods that just happen to be made without gluten. Therefore, even if the choices in your supermarket are limited, you can likely find some mainstream gluten-free foods that you can use until you have a chance to find a store with a larger variety of gluten-free foods and learn about gluten-free options offered by mail-order companies.

Many varieties of grain foods are made without gluten-containing ingredients. The following list includes examples and notes brands for some gluten-free products typically carried by supermarkets. Always check labels carefully and buy grain foods that are labeled gluten-free whenever possible.

- Ready-to-eat breakfast cereal: Labeled gluten-free varieties are available from General Mills (many types of Chex cereal), Kellogg's (Rice Krispies—there are two types so make sure you choose the product labeled gluten-free), and Post (types of Pebbles cereal).
- Plain brown rice.
- Plain enriched white rice.
- Plain specialty rice, such as basmati and jasmine.
- Rice cakes: Labeled gluten-free rice cakes are available from Quaker and Lundberg.
- Rice crackers: Labeled gluten-free crackers are available from KA-ME.
- Rice noodles: Labeled gluten-free noodles are available from Annie Chun's.
- Corn tortillas: Labeled gluten-free tortillas are available from Mission Foods.
- Taco shells: Some Ortega taco shells are labeled gluten-free.
- Unseasoned corn tortilla chips: Labeled gluten-free chips are available from Lay's.
- Grits.
- Plain popcorn.
- Polenta.
- Quinoa: Labeled gluten-free quinoa is available from Ancient Harvest (Quinoa Corporation).
- Baking mixes: Labeled gluten-free mixes are available from Betty Crocker.
- Pancake mixes: Labeled gluten-free mixes are available from Bisquick.

Gluten-Free Eating with Foods from the Supermarket

The following examples of gluten-free meals and snacks can be made with foods from your local supermarket. For more ideas, see the Sample Menu Ideas on page 22.

Breakfast

- Gluten-free rice cakes with peanut butter and sliced banana
- Omelet with low-fat cheddar cheese and diced red and green bell peppers
- Plain low-fat yogurt with blueberries and plain sliced almonds

Lunch

- Gluten-free corn tortilla topped with chickpeas, tomatoes, low-fat Swiss cheese, and herbs
- Nachos made with gluten-free tortilla chips, black beans, diced vegetables, gluten-free salsa, and low-fat Monterey Jack cheese
- Chicken salad served over greens with gluten-free rice crackers

Dinner

- Tacos made with gluten-free corn tortillas filled with chicken, fish, or beans, and sautéed vegetables
- Shrimp and vegetable stir-fry (made with gluten-free tamari, gluten-free soy sauce, or oil and spices) served over brown rice, enriched white rice, gluten-free rice noodles, or gluten-free quinoa
- Grilled salmon, baked potato topped with sautéed mushrooms, and salad with oil and vinegar

Snacks

- Trail mix made with plain almonds, raisins, and plain sunflower seeds
- Gluten-free rice crackers with peanut butter and marmalade
- Sliced apples and low-fat cheddar cheese
- Sliced banana and peanut butter

Sources of Gluten-Free Products

You can buy the following products through mail-order companies, at natural food stores, and at supermarkets with natural food sections or a large selection of gluten-free products. (Always check labels! Some manufacturers also make food products that are not gluten-free.) Ask your local natural food store or supermarket to carry your favorite gluten-free foods if you cannot readily find them.

Most manufacturers have store locator services on their websites to help you find stores in your area that carry their products. The companies listed here are provided for convenience only. This is not a complete listing of available gluten-free products.

Grains and Flours

There are many types of gluten-free grains, such as rice, corn, buckwheat, quinoa, teff, oats, and millet. You can also buy gluten-free flours made from these grains or from potato, amaranth, sorghum, beans, or nuts. Look, too, for specialty flour blends designed for baking gluten-free foods. The following are some of the many companies that carry gluten-free products. **Note**: Not all products carried by some of these companies are gluten-free. Read labels carefully.

Authentic Foods
www.authenticfoods.com
Phone: 800-806-4737

Avena Foods
www.avenafoods.com
Phone: 866-461-3663

The Birkett Mills
www.thebirkettmills.com
Phone: 315-536-3311

Bob's Red Mill
www.bobsredmill.com
Phone: 800-349-2173

Cream Hill Estates
www.creamhillestates.com
Phone: 866-727-3628

Gluten-Free Harvest
www.glutenfreeoats.com
Phone: 888-941-9922

Quinoa Corporation
www.quinoa.net
Phone: 301-217-8125

The Teff Company
www.teffco.com
Phone: 888-822-2221

Bread Products

You have many gluten-free bread and bread product choices (both ready-made and mixes), including sandwich breads, rolls, bagels, muffins, pizza crusts, and waffles. The following are some of the many companies that carry gluten-free products. **Note**: Not all products carried by some of these companies are gluten-free. Read labels carefully.

Dr. Schar
www.schar.com/us
Phone: 201-355-8470

Kinnikinnick Foods
www.kinnikinnick.com
Phone: 877-503-4466

Ener-G Foods
www.ener-g.com
Phone: 800-331-5222

Nature's Path
www.naturespath.com
Phone: 866-972-6879

Gillian's Foods
www.gilliansfoods.com
Phone: 781-586-0086

Rudi's Gluten-Free Bakery
www.rudisglutenfree.com
Phone: 877-293-0876

Gluten-Free Creations
www.glutenfreecreations.com
Phone: 602-522-0659

Udi's
www.udisglutenfree.com
Phone: 201-421-3970

Glutino
www.glutino.com
Phone: 201-421-3970

Van's International Foods
www.vansfoods.com
Phone: 323-585-8923

Pastas

A wide variety of gluten-free pastas—including those made from rice, corn, potato, millet, buckwheat, soy, amaranth, and quinoa—are available from the following companies. **Note**: Not all products carried by some of these companies are gluten-free. Read labels carefully.

Ancient Harvest (manufactured by Quinoa Corporation)
www.quinoa.net
Phone: 310-217-8125

Annie's Homegrown
www.annies.com
Phone: 800-288-1089

DeBole's
www.deboles.com
Phone: 800-434-4246

Heartland Pasta
www.heartlandpasta.com

Jovial Pasta
www.jovialfoods.com
Phone: 877-642-0644

Lundberg Family Farms
www.lundberg.com
Phone: 530-538-3500

Mrs. Leeper's
www.mrsleepers.com
Phone: 973-338-0300

Orgran
www.orgran.com

Pastariso and Pastato
(manufactured by Maplegrove
Gluten-Free Foods)
www.maplegrovefoods.com
Phone: 909-823-8230

Tinkyada (manufactured by Food
Directions, Inc.)
www.tinkyada.com

Breakfast Cereals

A large variety of gluten-free cereals, including those made from corn, rice, oats, sorghum, and buckwheat, are available. In addition to the mainstream manufacturers that produce gluten-free cereal, like General Mills, Kellogg's, and Post, the companies listed here carry gluten-free products. **Note**: Not all products manufactured by some of these companies are gluten-free. Read labels carefully.

Barbara's Bakery
www.barbaras.com
Phone: 800-343-0590

Bob's Red Mill
www.bobsredmill.com
Phone: 800-349-2173

Enjoy Life Natural Brands
www.enjoylifefoods.com
Phone: 888-503-6569

Erewhon (manufactured by
Attune Foods)
www.attunefoods.com

Nature's Path and **Envirokidz**
www.naturespath.com
Phone: 866-880-7284

Pocono (manufactured by the
Birkett Mills)
www.thebirkettmills.com
Phone: 315-536-3311

Gluten-Free Supplements

C-liac Vitality Packs
www.glutenfreevitamins.com
Phone: 888-861-7979

Freeda
www.freedavitamins.com
Phone: 800-777-3737

Country Life
www.country-life.com
Phone: 800-645-5768

Pioneer Nutritionals
www.pioneernutritional.com
Phone: 800-660-7742

Gluten-Free Oats

Avena Foods
www.avenafoods.com
Phone: 866-461-3663

Gluten Free Harvest
www.glutenfreeoats.com
Phone: 888-941-9922

Cream Hill Estates
www.creamhillestates.com
Phone: 866-727-3628

Low-Gluten Altar Breads

Benedictine Sisters of Perpetual Adoration
www.benedictinesisters.org
Phone: 800-223-2772

Ener-G Foods, Inc.
www.ener-g.com
Phone: 800-331-5222

Gluten-Free Matzo

Lakewood Matzoh Bakery
www.lakewoodmatzoh.com
Phone: 732-364-8757

Yehuda Matzo
www.yehudamatzos.com
Note: Imported to the United States during Passover.

Gluten-Free Beer

Anheuser-Busch
www.anheuser-busch.com
Phone: 800-342-5283
Carries gluten-free Redbridge beer
made from sorghum.

Lakefront Brewery
www.lakefrontbrewery.com
Phone: 414-372-8800
Carries gluten-free New Grist beer
made from sorghum and rice.

Bard's Tale Beer
www.bardsbeer.com
Phone: 877-440-2337
Carries gluten-free beer made from
malted sorghum.

Sample Menu Ideas

There are gluten-free versions of almost all wheat-based products.
Therefore, a gluten-free diet does not have to be much different from a
wheat-based diet. The following examples of meals and snacks illustrate
the variety of food products available at natural food stores and through
mail-order companies, as well as at some supermarkets with large gluten-
free food sections.

Breakfast

- Gluten-free waffles topped with walnuts, blueberries, and pure
  maple syrup
- Whole grain or fortified gluten-free cereal mixed with low-fat
  yogurt
- Poached egg on whole grain or enriched gluten-free toast

Lunch

- Tuna melt made with a gluten-free bagel or gluten-free English
  muffin topped with tuna salad and melted low-fat cheese, served
  with gluten-free rice noodle soup
- Mixed salad with leafy greens, tomato, green beans, corn, kidney
  beans, and avocado topped with oil and vinegar and gluten-free
  croutons

- Cheese quesadilla made with gluten-free corn tortillas, with fresh gluten-free tomato salsa and guacamole

Dinner

- Gluten-free pasta with pesto and chickpeas
- Pizza made with gluten-free pizza crust, topped with tomato sauce, low-fat mozzarella, and vegetables
- Chicken and vegetable stir-fry served over gluten-free quinoa, sprinkled with gluten-free soy sauce

Snacks

- Gluten-free muffin and low-fat milk
- Gluten-free pretzels and peanut butter
- Gluten-free snack bar

Avoiding Cross-Contact at Home

Cross-contact can occur whenever a gluten-free food comes in contact with a gluten-containing food. To lessen the chances of cross-contact at home, follow these tips:

- Store gluten-free products, especially those that make crumbs (such as bread, cookies, and crackers), separately from gluten-containing products. If you can, store gluten-free foods in a separate cupboard. If that is not practical, store gluten-free foods on a shelf **above** gluten-containing foods.
- Store gluten-free flours, gluten-free baking mixes, and baking and cooking ingredients that you use only for gluten-free food preparation (for example, spices, baking soda, baking powder) separately from gluten-containing flours, mixes, and ingredients. Again, a separate cupboard for gluten-free flours and mixes is best. If that is not practical, store gluten-free flours, mixes, and other ingredients on a shelf **above** gluten-containing flours.
- Store gluten-free flours inside zippered plastic bags to prevent cross-contact.

- After preparing foods that contain gluten, wash your hands before preparing gluten-free foods.

- Designate certain appliances (for example, toaster, bread machine, and food processor) for use only with gluten-free products. If that is not practical, clean your appliances well between uses.

- Use reusable toaster bags in the toaster or toaster oven. They may be mail-ordered from Amazon (www.amazon.com).

- Use separate serving utensils and food preparation tools, such as pasta tongs and cutting boards, when preparing both gluten-free and gluten-containing foods. Or, prepare the gluten-free foods first.

- To prevent contamination of butter, peanut butter, jelly, condiments, and other spreadables with gluten-containing bread crumbs, buy two of each product and label one for gluten-free use only. Or, have a "no double-dipping rule" for knives, spoons, and other utensils.

- When grilling hot dog buns or rolls, grill the gluten-free portions first.

- When frying breaded products, cook all gluten-free foods first.

- When food is served "family style" at the table, use separate serving utensils for the gluten-free foods.

Tip: Many recipes use gluten-free flours, but you can also adapt your favorite **wheat flour–based** recipes. Just use ¾ cup of a gluten-free flour (such as brown rice flour) and ¼ cup of a gluten-free starch (such as cornstarch) for every 1 cup of wheat flour called for in a recipe. For information on gluten-free cookbooks, see page 42.

Tips for Eating Away from Home

Deciding what foods to eat when an ingredients list is not available can be a challenge. However, a gluten-free diet should not keep you from enjoying a restaurant meal, eating at a friend's house, or traveling. The following tips may help:

- When traveling, pack basic, nonperishable gluten-free grain foods, such as cereal, bread, rice cakes, pasta, snack bars, and crackers.
- When eating at other people's homes, let them know about your dietary restrictions. Help your host by bringing a gluten-free dish for everyone to enjoy.
- When eating at restaurants, bring your own gluten-free bread, rolls, or pasta (depending on the type of restaurant). Many restaurants will substitute the customer's gluten-free food when making a sandwich or pasta dish. Remember to make sure that the restaurant takes steps to prevent cross-contact with its wheat-based products.
- The "safest" choices to order at a restaurant are plain foods without added breading, sauces, marinades, or gravies. One example of a gluten-free restaurant meal is broiled scallops with lemon, a baked potato with butter and chives, and steamed broccoli.
- Before going to a restaurant, call ahead to speak with someone familiar with menu ingredients, such as the chef. Explain your dietary restrictions and discuss the available gluten-free options.
- Use caution when eating at restaurants where cross-contact may be a concern.
  - Before ordering French fries, ask if they are coated with flour or cooked in the same oil used to fry breaded foods that are not gluten-free, such as onion rings. If they are, don't order the French fries. Tortilla chips, corn tortillas, or taco shells may be fried in a shared fryer, too.
  - Also, ask if your food will be cooked on the same grill surface as breaded products that are not gluten-free, such as hamburger buns. If the same surface is used, ask that a portion of the grill be cleaned before your food is cooked or that a separate pan be used.
- Many restaurants now offer gluten-free menus, including the chains Legal Sea Foods (www.legalseafoods.com), Outback Steakhouse (www.outback.com), and P.F. Chang's (www.pfchangs.com).

Find more tips for eating gluten-free when away from home in the book *The Essential Gluten-Free Restaurant Guide*, by Triumph Dining, and in the free iPhone and Android app *Find Me Gluten Free*. See the Additional Sources of Information in this booklet for more information.

How to Get the Nutrients You Need

A gluten-free diet should be based on whole grain and enriched grain foods, as well as fresh, frozen, unprocessed, or lightly processed vegetables, fruits, milk products (or nondairy equivalents such as soymilk fortified with calcium and vitamin D), and protein foods (lean meats, poultry, fish, dried beans, nuts, seeds, and eggs).

The USDA developed MyPlate to help you choose foods that meet your daily nutrient needs. MyPlate provides recommended daily amounts from the grain, fruit, vegetable, protein, and dairy groups.

For the dairy group, the amount you need depends on your age. The amounts you need from the other four food groups depend on your calorie needs, which are based on your age, gender, and activity level. For example, women between the ages of 31 to 50 years who get less than 30 minutes of moderate exercise a day should eat the following amounts each day:

- 6 ounces of grains, at least half of which should be whole grain
- 1½ cups of fruit
- 2½ cups of vegetables
- 3 cups of fat-free or low-fat milk (or a nondairy equivalent)
- 5 ounce equivalents of meat, fish, dried beans, and other protein foods

For information on the amount of food you should be eating each day and information on what counts as a serving, visit the MyPlate website (www. ChooseMyPlate.gov) or ask your doctor or registered dietitian (RD).

B Vitamins, Iron, and Fiber

Whole grain, enriched, and fortified varieties of breads, cereals, rice, and pasta contain essential nutrients, including iron and several B vitamins (thiamin, riboflavin, niacin, and folate). Whole grain foods are also rich in fiber.

In the United States, most refined wheat flours, wheat-based breads, and wheat-based pasta products are enriched with iron and B vitamins. Most breakfast cereals are fortified with those nutrients as well as others.

When a whole grain, such as brown rice, is milled to make a refined product, such as white rice, the outer layers of the grain are removed. Fiber and many vitamins and minerals are found in the outer layers. Therefore, refined, unenriched grain products contain less of these nutrients than whole grain products. Enrichment of refined grain products replaces vitamins and minerals lost during the milling process. However, enrichment does not replace the fiber that was removed.

Unfortunately, many gluten-free grain foods contain refined corn or refined rice flour and/or starch instead of whole grains. They also tend to not be enriched. As a result, they may not provide the same amounts of nutrients as wheat-containing foods. To get more B vitamins, iron, and fiber in your diet, follow the tips in the next sections.

Choose Whole Grain Gluten-Free Foods Instead of Refined Foods

Check ingredients lists on product labels, and choose whole grain gluten-free foods made from whole corn, brown rice, sorghum, millet, wild rice, or teff. Ingredients are listed according to weight from the highest amount to the lowest amount. Ideally, a gluten-free whole grain is the first ingredient in the list.

Table 1 (on page 28) illustrates the nutritional differences between whole grain and refined products. As you can see, the brown rice flour provides more B vitamins (thiamin, riboflavin, niacin, and folate), iron, and fiber than the white rice flour.

Table 1. Nutrient Content of 100 Grams of White and Brown Rice Flour

Nutrient	White Rice Flour	Brown Rice Flour
Thiamin	0.14 milligrams (mg)	0.44 mg
Riboflavin	0.02 mg	0.08 mg
Niacin	2.59 mg	6.34 mg
Folate	4 micrograms (µg) Dietary Folate Equivalents (DFE)	16 µg DFE
Iron	0.35 mg	1.98 mg
Fiber	2.4 grams (g)	4.6 g

Source: USDA Nutrient Database for Standard Reference, Release 26. www.nal.usda.gov/fnic.

Choose Enriched Gluten-Free Grain Foods Instead of Refined, Unenriched Foods

Manufacturers of gluten-free grain foods that offer products enriched with B vitamins and iron include:

- Ener-G Foods, Gluten-Free Creations, Glutino, and Kinnikinnick Foods for ready-made bread products
- Enjoy Life Natural Brands for ready-made granola cereals
- Glutino for baking mixes
- Maplegrove Gluten-Free Foods for gluten-free Pastato pasta
- General Mills, Kellogg's, and Post for gluten-free cereals fortified with several vitamins and minerals

Table 2 illustrates the nutritional differences between enriched and unenriched refined products. As you can see, the enriched corn flour provides more B vitamins and iron than the unenriched corn flour.

Table 2. Nutrient Content of 100 Grams of Enriched and Unenriched Corn Flour

Nutrient	Enriched Corn Flour	Unenriched Corn Flour
Thiamin	1.48 milligrams (mg)	0.07 mg
Riboflavin	0.81 mg	0.06 mg
Niacin	9.93 mg	2.66 mg
Folate	335 micrograms (µg) Dietary Folate Equivalents (DFE)	48 µg DFE
Iron	7.49 mg	0.91 mg

Source: USDA Nutrient Database for Standard Reference, Release 26. www.nal.usda.gov/fnic.

Eat More Gluten-Free Grain Products Made from Buckwheat, Amaranth, and Quinoa

Buckwheat, amaranth, and quinoa are good sources of iron, fiber, and some B vitamins. Examples of products made from these plant foods include buckwheat hot cereal, amaranth bread, amaranth flatbread, and quinoa pasta.

Eat More Nongrain Sources of B Vitamins, Iron, and Fiber

Table 3 lists many nongrain foods that supply B vitamins (thiamin, riboflavin, niacin, and folate), iron, and fiber.

Table 3. Nongrain Sources of B Vitamins, Iron, and Fiber

Nutrient	Food Sources
Thiamin	Lean cuts of fresh pork
	Legumes (black beans, split peas, lentils)
	Nuts (Brazil, pistachio, pine nuts)
	Fish (salmon, tuna)
	Soymilk

continues

Table 3. Nongrain Sources of B Vitamins, Iron, and Fiber, *cont'd*

Nutrient, *cont'd*	Food Sources, *cont'd*
Riboflavin	Dairy products (yogurt, cottage cheese) Legumes (kidney beans, soybeans, black-eyed peas) Nuts (almonds) Green leafy vegetables (spinach) Mushrooms
Niacin	Poultry (turkey) Fish (fresh tuna, swordfish, halibut, salmon) Lean cuts of fresh pork Legumes (lentils, peanuts) Seeds (sunflower seeds)
Folate	Legumes (chickpeas, kidney beans, lentils, split peas) Green leafy vegetables (collard greens, turnip greens, spinach) Fruit juices (orange, tomato, pineapple)
Iron	Lean cuts of beef Poultry Seafood (clams, oysters) Legumes (white beans, lentils, kidney beans, split peas) Dried fruits (prunes, raisins, dates) and prune juice Green leafy vegetables (turnip greens, spinach) Other vegetables (green peas, cooked mushrooms, potatoes, pumpkin) Nuts and seeds (pine nuts, pumpkin seeds)
Fiber	All plant foods—fruits, vegetables, legumes (dried beans, peas, lentils), seeds, and nuts

Consider Taking a Gluten-Free Multivitamin and Mineral Supplement

You and your RD should decide whether you need a multivitamin and mineral supplement. Several gluten-free brands are available, including C-liac Vitality Packs, Country Life, Freeda, and Pioneer Nutritionals. Make sure that the supplement you choose contains all the vitamins and minerals in the amounts recommended by your RD.

Calcium and Lactose Intolerance

Some people newly diagnosed with celiac disease have a temporary form of lactose intolerance, called **secondary lactose intolerance**, which is caused by damage to the lining of the small intestine. Secondary lactose intolerance often goes away after the intestine heals in response to a gluten-free diet.

When you are lactose intolerant, your body does not make enough of the enzyme **lactase** to break down **lactose** (the sugar found in milk). When you drink milk or eat dairy foods, you may experience abdominal pain or bloating, gas, diarrhea, or nausea.

Milk and other dairy products are the major sources of calcium for most Americans. Your diet should contain adequate amounts of calcium for good bone health. If you are lactose intolerant, you can get calcium from many nondairy foods, including:

- Grains, such as amaranth and teff
- Orange juice with added calcium
- Soymilk with added calcium
- Leafy green vegetables, such as spinach and collards
- Legumes, such as white beans and black-eyed peas
- Fish, such as salmon and sardines (canned with bones)
- Soybeans
- Tofu prepared with calcium sulfate

You may also be able to eat dairy foods with low levels of lactose, including:

- Lactose-free milk, such as Lactaid brand (www.lactaid.com)
- Aged natural cheese, such as cheddar and Swiss
- Yogurt with active cultures

Some people take lactase enzyme supplements before eating to help them tolerate the lactose in dairy foods. These supplements are available in a variety of forms, including tablets. Make sure the supplements you take are gluten-free. According to the Lactaid website (www.lactaid.com),

Lactaid brand Fast Act caplets, Lactaid Fast Act chewables, and Lactaid brand Original Strength caplets do not contain gluten.

For more information on lactose intolerance, see the National Digestive Diseases Information Center Clearinghouse Website: www.niddk.nih.gov/health/digest/pubs/lactose/lactose.htm.

Frequently Asked Questions

What is gluten?

For the definition of gluten, turn to page 1.

What is meant by the term "gluten-free"?

A food can be labeled gluten-free, if:

- It is naturally free of gluten, **or**
- It is made without the gluten-containing grains wheat, barley, or rye, and it is made without ingredients from these grains that have not been processed to remove gluten (for example, wheat flour).

A gluten-free food also must contain less than 20 ppm of gluten.

Where can I find more information about U.S. labeling rules?

For more information about the FDA rule on gluten-free labeling, see:

- Food Labeling: Gluten-Free Labeling of Foods (http://tinyurl.com/q9l4ykn)
- Questions and Answers: Gluten-Free Food Labeling Rule Final (http://tinyurl.com/q6zezf7)

For more information on gluten-free labeling of USDA-regulated foods, see the Gluten-Free Dietitian's newsletter page (www.glutenfreedietitian. com/newsletter/2009/11/11/labeling-of-usda-regulated-foods-straight-from-the-usda).

For more information on the TTB's rules for the gluten-free labeling of alcoholic beverages, see the Gluten-Free Dietitian's newsletter page (www. glutenfreedietitian.com/newsletter/gluten-free-labeling-of-alcoholic-beverages-update).

For more information on FALCPA, see the FDA's online page "Food Allergen Labeling and Consumer Protection Act of 2004 Questions and Answers" (www.fda.gov/Food/GuidanceRegulation/Guidance DocumentsRegulatoryInformation/Allergens/ucm106890.htm).

Can other family members safely follow a gluten-free diet if they don't have celiac disease?

Eating healthy gluten-free foods will not harm people who do not have celiac disease. However, it is not a good idea to follow a strict gluten-free diet when it is not medically prescribed because the diet would unnecessarily restrict food choices, which may make it more difficult to get enough of certain vitamins and minerals.

Note: First- and second-degree relatives of persons who have been diagnosed with celiac disease are more likely than the general population to have celiac disease. They should speak with their doctor about being tested for celiac disease before following a gluten-free diet.

Can I occasionally eat gluten-containing foods?

No! You should follow a strict gluten-free diet and not eat any gluten-containing foods. Eating even small amounts of gluten can damage the small intestine. The FDA defines a gluten-free food as one that contains less than 20 ppm of gluten. A 1-ounce slice of gluten-free bread with almost 20 ppm of gluten contains a little more than ½ milligram of gluten. In contrast, if you cut a 1-ounce slice of wheat bread into 7,030 pieces, each of those tiny crumbs contains the same amount of gluten as the entire slice of gluten-free bread.

When grocery shopping, am I limited to foods and beverages that are labeled gluten-free?

No! The FDA allows any naturally gluten-free food (for example, a bag of raw carrots or bottled water) to be labeled gluten-free as long as it contains less than 20 ppm gluten. However, many naturally gluten-free foods and beverages (for example, bottled water) have little or no risk of cross-contact with gluten-containing grains. In these low-risk cases, it is generally safe to buy the food or beverage even if it does not have a gluten-free label.

Other foods have a much higher risk of cross-contact (for example, grains and flours). In these higher-risk cases, it is advisable to choose foods labeled gluten-free.

> **Note:** The next three questions deal with ingredients that can be derived from wheat. Under the Food Allergen Labeling and Consumer Protection Act (FALCPA), if a food is regulated by the FDA and it includes an ingredient that contains wheat protein, the word "wheat" must be listed on the food label, either in the ingredients list or Contains statement. However, the FDA's gluten-free labeling rule allows for some ingredients derived from wheat as long as they have been processed to remove gluten and the final food product contains less than 20 ppm of gluten. All foods labeled gluten-free may be a part of your diet.

Can I eat foods that contain wheat starch?

The answer depends on the specific food product.
- If a food contains wheat starch and it **is** labeled gluten-free, you may eat it. Under the FDA's gluten-free labeling rule, a food may contain wheat starch and be labeled gluten-free as long as the final food product contains less than 20 ppm of gluten.
- If a product contains wheat starch and it **is not** labeled gluten-free, you should **not** eat it. The food containing the wheat starch may contain 20 ppm or more of gluten.

Can I eat foods that contain modified food starch, starch, or dextrin?

If modified food starch, starch, or dextrin is included in the ingredients list of a food regulated by the FDA and you do not see the word "wheat" in either the ingredients list or the Contains statement, these ingredients do **not** contain wheat protein.

You can safely eat food products that contain modified food starch, starch, and dextrin derived from wheat when the products are labeled gluten-free. This is because the FDA allows wheat-based modified food starch, wheat-based starch, and wheat-based dextrin to be included in foods labeled gluten-free as long as the final food product contains less than 20 ppm of gluten.

If a food product that contains modified food starch, starch, or dextrin includes the word "wheat"in either the ingredients list or Contains statement, **and** the product is not labeled gluten-free, you should **not** eat the food.

Note: If you see the single word "starch" in the ingredients list of an FDA-regulated food product that means the product contains cornstarch.

Can I eat foods that contain maltodextrin, glucose syrup, or caramel?

If maltodextrin, glucose syrup, or caramel is included in the ingredients list of a food regulated by the FDA and you do not see the word "wheat" in either the ingredients list or the Contains statement, these ingredients do **not** contain wheat protein.

You can eat food products that contain the ingredients maltodextrin, glucose syrup, or caramel derived from wheat when the products are labeled gluten-free. This is because the FDA allows wheat-based maltodextrin, wheat-based glucose syrup, and wheat-based caramel color to be included in foods labeled gluten-free as long as the final food product contains less than 20 ppm of gluten.

Even if maltodextrin, glucose syrup, or caramel color is made from wheat, these ingredients are considered gluten-free. The amount of gluten they contain is highly unlikely to cause a final food product to contain 20 ppm or more gluten.

What is an allergen advisory statement?

Allergen advisory statements are voluntary statements that some manufacturers place on food labels to alert consumers to food processing practices. Examples include "processed in a facility that processes foods containing wheat" and "may contain wheat." These statements are not currently defined by any federal regulation. Because these statements are voluntary, some manufacturers use them and others do not.

How can foods be labeled gluten-free when they contain an allergen advisory statement for wheat?

Foods labeled gluten-free must contain less than 20 ppm of gluten, regardless of whether the gluten comes from ingredients or cross-contact. Refer to the section on cross-contact on page 13 of this booklet for more information.

Can I eat foods that contain the ingredient "natural flavor"?

If a food containing natural flavor does not include the words "wheat," "barley," "rye," "oats," "malt," or "brewer's yeast" in the ingredients list, and it does not list wheat in a Contains statement, the natural flavor is most likely free of gluten.

Can I eat oats?

Oats are a naturally gluten-free grain. However, they can be contaminated with wheat, barley, or rye when they are harvested, transported, stored, milled, and/or processed, especially if the same equipment is used for oats and the gluten-containing grains. As a consequence, people with celiac disease should eat only oats and oat products that are labeled gluten-free.

While most people with celiac disease can eat moderate amounts of oats that are labeled gluten-free, there is very limited scientific evidence that the prolamin (protein) avenin in oats may cause intestinal damage in a minority of persons with celiac disease.

The decision to include oats in your diet is one that you should make with your doctor and RD. If you decide to include oats in your diet, you should:

- Eat only oats that are labeled gluten-free. (See Sources of Gluten-

Free Products on page 21.)

- Limit the amount of dry oats you eat to 50 grams per day. That amount is about ½ cup of dry, whole-grain rolled oats or ¼ cup of dry, steel-cut oats.
- Contact your RD or physician if you experience any gastrointestinal symptoms after adding oats to your diet.

Can I eat spelt, emmer, einkorn, or khorasan?

No. These are all types of wheat and should not be part of a gluten-free diet.

Can I eat buckwheat?

Yes. Buckwheat is **not** a type of wheat and may safely be included in a gluten-free diet.

Can I eat distilled vinegar?

Yes. Although distilled vinegar is made from a grain mash that may include wheat, barley, or rye, it is safe to include in a gluten-free diet. The process of distillation should remove all protein from the final product.

Can I eat malt vinegar?

No. Malt vinegar contains barley and should **not** be eaten on a gluten-free diet.

If I choose to drink alcoholic beverages, what should I know about wine, beer, and distilled alcohol?

Wine is fermented from grapes and is considered gluten-free.

When choosing a beer, check the label. Most beers are made with malted barley and are not gluten-free. However, labeled gluten-free beers made using a substitute for malted barley, such as sorghum, are available (see page 22).

Some beers made with malted barley have undergone a process to remove gluten. These products may **not** be labeled gluten-free. However, under current TTB policy, they may be labeled "Processed or treated or crafted to remove gluten." The labels on these beers must also state: "Product fermented from grains containing gluten and processed or treated or crafted to remove gluten. The gluten content of this product cannot be verified, and this product may contain gluten."

Pure distilled alcoholic beverages (for example, gin and vodka) are considered safe for people with celiac disease. Although wheat, barley, or rye may be used to produce pure distilled alcoholic beverages, the distillation process should prevent gluten from remaining in the alcohol.

Nevertheless, distilled alcoholic beverages made from gluten-containing grains or any ingredients derived from these grains may **not** be labeled gluten-free. Instead, these products may be labeled "Processed or treated or crafted to remove gluten" **if** the product has been processed to remove all or some of the gluten. The label must also state, "This product was distilled from grains containing gluten, which removed some or all of the gluten. The gluten content of this product cannot be verified, and this product may contain gluten."

Additional Sources of Information

The resources listed here provide useful information on celiac disease and the gluten-free diet.

National Support Groups and Patient Advocacy Groups

American Celiac Disease Alliance
www.americanceliac.org
Phone: (703) 622-3331
E-mail: info@americanceliac.org

Celiac Disease Foundation (CDF)
www.celiac.org
Phone: 818-716-1513
E-mail: info@celiac.org

Celiac Sprue Association (CSA)
www.csaceliacs.org
Phone: 877-272-4272
E-mail: celiacs@csaceliacs.org

The Gluten Intolerance Group (GIG)
www.gluten.net
Phone: 253-833-6655
E-mail: CustomerService@gluten.net

National Foundation for Celiac Awareness
www.celiaccentral.org
Phone: 215-325-1306
E-mail: info@celiaccentral.org

Celiac Disease Medical Centers

Celiac Center at Beth Israel Deaconess Medical Center (Boston)
www.bidmc.org/celiaccenter
Phone: 617-667-1272

The Celiac Center at Paoli Hospital (Paoli, PA)
www.mainlinehealth.org/paoliceliac
Phone: 866-225-5654

Celiac Disease Center at Columbia University (New York City)
www.celiacdiseasecenter.columbia.edu
Phone: 212-342-4529

Celiac Disease Clinic at Mayo Clinic
www.mayoclinic.org/celiac-disease

Celiac Disease Program at Boston Children's Hospital
www.childrenshospital.org/
health-topics/conditions/c/
celiac-disease
Phone: 617-355-2127

Celiac Group at the University of Virginia Health Systems (Charlottesville)
www.healthsystem.virginia.edu/
internet/digestive-health/patient
care.cfm
Phone: 434-924-2959

Center for Celiac Research and Treatment at Massachusetts General Hospital (Boston)
Website: www.massgeneral.org/
children/services/treatment
programs.aspx?id=1723
Phone: 617-724-8476

Kogan Celiac Center (Livingston, NJ)
www.saintbarnabas.com/services/
celiac/index.html
Phone: 888-724-7123

Stanford Celiac Sprue Management Clinic (Stanford, CA)
http://stanfordhospital.org/clinics
medServices/clinics/gastroenter
ology/celiacSprue.html
Phone: 650-723-6961

UCLA Celiac Disease Program (Los Angeles)
http://gastro.ucla.edu/body.
cfm?id=20
Phone: Please see website for individual physician contact numbers

University of Chicago Celiac Disease Program
www.uchospitals.edu/specialties/
celiac
Phone: 888-824-0200

Wm. K. Warren Medical Research Center for Celiac Disease (San Diego)
http://celiaccenter.ucsd.edu
Phone: 858-822-1022

Magazines

Allergic Living
http://allergicliving.com
Phone: 888-771-7747
E-mail: info@allergicliving.com
Magazine for people with asthma, allergies, and gluten-related disorders.

Gluten-Free Living
www.glutenfreeliving.com
Phone: 800-437-5828
E-mail: info@glutenfreeliving.com
Magazine for people with celiac disease and dermatitis herpetiformis.

Delight Gluten-Free
www.delightglutenfree.com
Phone: 800-305-6964 ext. 101
E-mail: info@delightglutenfree.com
Magazine for people with food sensitivities and allergies.

Living Without
www.livingwithout.com
Phone: 800-474-8614
E-mail: Editor@LivingWithout.com
Magazine for people with food allergies, intolerances, and sensitivities, including celiac disease.

Websites

Academy of Nutrition and Dietetics: www.eatright.org
Use the Search function on this site to find information on celiac disease. You can also use the site to find a registered dietitian in your area.

Celiac Now: www.celiacnow.org
This site teaches the nutritional and medical management of celiac disease and the gluten-free diet. Each topic is divided into three levels (from introductory to complex) to appeal to a variety of different readers.

Dietary Guidelines for Americans, 2010:
www.health.gov/dietaryguidelines
This site posts the federal dietary guidelines, which are updated every 5 years.

Food Allergen Labeling and Consumer Protection Act of 2004 (FALCPA):
www.fda.gov/food/guidanceregulation/guidancedocumentsregulatory information/allergens/ucm106187.htm
This webpage posts the FALCPA law.

Food and Drug Administration Gluten-Free Labeling of Foods:
www.fda.gov/Food/GuidanceRegulation/GuidanceDocumentsRegulatory
Information/Allergens/ucm362510.htm
This webpage links to many publications on gluten-free labeling.

Food and Nutrition Information Center: www.nal.usda.gov/fnic
This site links to a variety of nutrition resources.

Gluten Free Dietitian Newsletter:
www.glutenfreedietitian.com/newsletter
The newsletter has many articles on issues related to celiac disease, non-celiac gluten sensitivity, and the gluten-free diet.

Gluten Free Diet News: www.glutenfreediet.ca/ezsignup.php
The newsletter page of this site has an archive of past issues.

Gluten Free Drugs: www.glutenfreedrugs.com
This site lists gluten-free medications and supplements. ·

Gluten Free Watchdog: www.glutenfreewatchdog.org
This site provides independent testing of gluten-free foods.

MyPlate: www.ChooseMyPlate.gov
This site has information about nutrition and food groups. Site tools can help you plan how much to eat each day.

National Institutes of Health (NIH) Celiac Disease Awareness Campaign: http://celiac.nih.gov
This site has current science-based information on celiac disease.

NIH Consensus Development Conference on Celiac Disease:
http://consensus.nih.gov/2004/2004CeliacDisease118html.htm
This site, published in 2004, describes research on celiac disease.

Cookbooks

Thompson, Tricia, and Marlisa Brown. *Easy Gluten-Free: Expert Nutrition Advice with More than 100 Recipes.* Wiley; 2010, Houghton Mifflin Harcourt; 2013.

Credicott, Tammy. *The Healthy Gluten-Free Life: 200 Delicious Gluten-Free, Dairy-Free, Soy-Free and Egg-Free Recipes!* Victory Belt Publishing; 2012.

Fenster, Carol. *125 Gluten-Free and Vegetarian Recipes.* Penguin Group; 2011.

Fenster, Carol. *100 Best Gluten-Free Recipes.* Wiley; 2010.

Landolphi, Robert. *Quick-Fix Gluten Free.* Andrews McMeel Publishing; 2011.

O'Brien, Susan. *The Gluten-Free Vegan: 150 Delicious Gluten-Free, Animal-Free Recipes.* De Capo Press; 2007.

General Information Books

Adamson, Eve, and Tricia Thompson. *The Complete Idiot's Guide to Gluten-Free Eating.* Penguin; 2007.

Blumer, Ian, and Sheila Crowe. *Celiac Disease for Dummies.* Penguin; 2007.

Case, Shelley. *Gluten-Free Diet: A Comprehensive Resource Guide.* 5th edition. Case Nutrition Consulting; 2014. www.glutenfreediet.ca.

Dennis, Melinda, and Daniel Leffler. *Real Life with Celiac Disease: Troubleshooting and Thriving Gluten-Free.* AGA Press; 2010.

The Essential Gluten-Free Grocery Guide. 5th edition. Triumph Dining Gluten-Free Publishing; 2012.

The Essential Gluten-Free Restaurant Guide. 6th edition. Triumph Dining Gluten-Free Publishing. www.triumphdining.com.

Green, Peter HR, and Rory Jones. *Celiac Disease: A Hidden Epidemic.* Revised edition. William Morrow; 2010.

Thompson, Tricia. *The Gluten-Free Nutrition Guide.* McGraw-Hill; 2008.

Apps and Dining Cards

Find Me Gluten-Free

iPhone and Google app that identifies local restaurants and other businesses with gluten-free options.

Triumph Dining Cards: www.triumphdining.com

Printed dining cards and phone apps that you can use in restaurants to explain the gluten-free diet. Cards are available for different cuisines and in different languages.

Recipes

Learning how to cook gluten-free meals can be overwhelming, especially when you have been newly diagnosed with celiac disease. Here are a couple of recipes to get you started. To find more gluten-free recipes, refer to the Cookbooks section of Additional Sources of Information on page 42.

Turkey Meatloaf

    1 teaspoon vegetable oil

    1 ⅓ pounds ground turkey

    ½ cup cooked quinoa

    1 egg

    ½ teaspoon salt

    ⅛ teaspoon black pepper

    1 teaspoon garlic powder

    ½ teaspoon onion powder

    ⅓ cup ketchup

    ½ teaspoon dried oregano

    ½ teaspoon dried thyme leaves

    ½ cup finely chopped onion

    2 stalks celery, finely chopped

    4 pieces turkey bacon, cut in halves

Preheat the oven to 350 degrees. Lightly coat a 9 × 5-inch loaf pan with vegetable oil. In a large bowl, mix together the turkey, quinoa, egg, salt, pepper, garlic powder, onion powder, ketchup, oregano, thyme, onion, and celery. Fill the loaf pan with the turkey mixture and spread with a spatula. Arrange the turkey bacon on top of the meatloaf, placing one slice next to the other to cover the whole loaf. Bake uncovered for 55 to 65 minutes until cooked through and the meatloaf reaches an internal temperature of 165 degrees.

Serves 8 (1⅛-inch slices).

Adapted from *American Dietetic Association Easy Gluten-Free: Expert Nutrition Advice with More Than 100 Recipes* by Tricia Thompson, MS, RD, and Marlisa Brown, MS, RD, CDE, CDN. Copyright © 2010 by American Dietetic Association. Reprinted by permission of Houghton Mifflin Harcourt Publishing Company. All rights reserved.

Wild Rice Pilaf

  1 cup wild rice

  1 pound asparagus, cut into ¼-inch pieces

  2 tablespoons olive oil

  1 clove garlic, minced

  ½ cup chopped onion

  ½ cup chopped green pepper

  1 cup chopped mushrooms

  2 tomatoes, chopped

  ⅔ cup gluten-free Italian dressing

  ¼ cup sunflower seed kernels

Cook the rice according to package directions. Microwave the asparagus for 3 minutes, until just tender. Heat the oil in a large skillet over medium heat. Add the garlic, onion, and pepper, and sauté for 3 to 4 minutes until softened. Add the mushrooms and cook for 1 to 2 minutes longer. Add the asparagus, tomatoes, rice, and dressing. Cook for 3 to 4 minutes until heated through. Sprinkle with sunflower seeds and serve immediately, or let cool and serve cold.

Serves 10 (½ cup servings).